Rotator Cuff Repair

A GUIDE FOR PATIENTS

By

David N. Collins, MD
University of Arkansas for Medical Sciences
Little Rock, Arkansas

Medical Board Editor
Professor David Seligson, MD, FRCS
Vice-Chair of Orthopedic Surgery
and Chief of Fracture Service
University of Louisville School of Medicine

231 Market Place, No. 331, San Ramon, CA 94583 (800) HIN-1947

ISBN 1-885274-52-1

MADE IN THE U.S.A.

About the Author

Dr. Collins is a clinical faculty member of the Department of Orthopaedic Surgery at the University of Arkansas for Medical Sciences in Little Rock. A member of the American Shoulder and Elbow Surgeons, Dr. Collins is actively involved in physician education and clinical research. He has published scientific articles and chapters on a wide range of orthopedic topics.

Medical Consultants: Warren D. King, MD, Lana S. Sandahl, DC

Staff Editors: Leah Dible, Jeffery Stoia

Production Manager: Mary F. Gadbois

Illustrators: Peg Magovern, Walter Denn, John Rutherford, Andree Policicchio, Todd Leonardo

We hope you will gain much benefit from this booklet.

HIN, Inc. The Health Information Network

TABLE OF CONTENTS

INTRODUCTION

The shoulder has the widest range of motion of any joint in the human body. Usually, the shoulder can safely perform all we ask of it. However, great stresses at the shoulder joint increase its chance for injury.

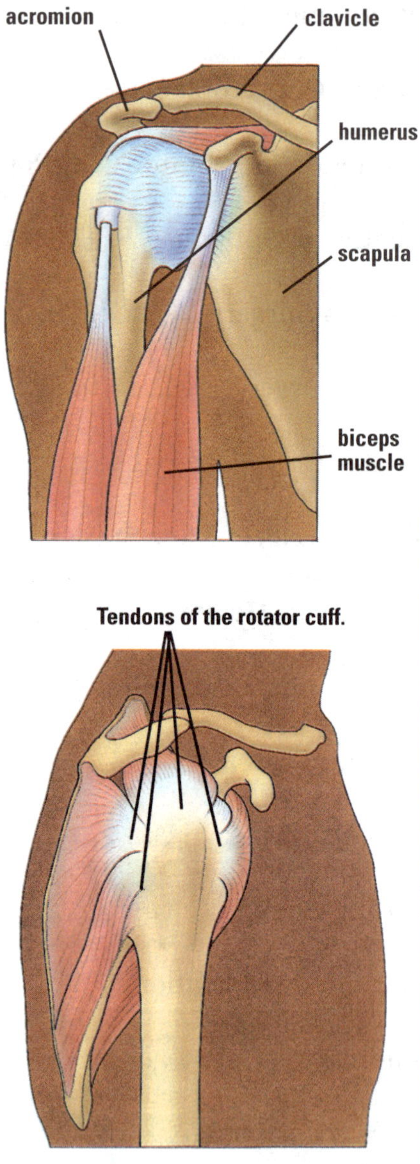

Anatomy of the shoulder.

What Is the Rotator Cuff?

The **rotator cuff** is the name given to a group of four tendons that connect four short muscles of the shoulder blade to the upper arm bone (**humerus**). A **tendon** is tough, stringy tissue that connects muscle to bone. These muscles help to control overhead arm movement. They also help to keep the shoulder stable.

ROTATOR CUFF PROBLEMS

Problems with the rotator cuff can vary in severity. Problems can be caused by tears in a rotator cuff tendon, or more commonly, by a condition called **impingement.**

Impingement

Shoulder dislocation, fracture, or a violent injury can cause a tear in the rotator cuff. Most tears, however, are due to impingement.

Impingement is a disorder of the shoulder caused by a narrowing of the space in which the rotator cuff can move. This increases the pressure between the rotator cuff and the bone.

- This can result from aging or, less commonly, an accident. Weakness of the tendons or muscles of the rotator cuff allows the upper arm bone to move up toward the **acromion** (part of the **scapula,** or shoulder blade), narrowing the space between them.
- Some people naturally have less space for the rotator cuff. The acromion may be shaped in a way that "pinches" the rotator cuff when the arm is raised.
- The rotator cuff may become damaged from the increased pressure as it rubs against the **acromion**.

A tear in the rotator cuff can develop immediately or soon after a traumatic injury to the shoulder. It may take months or years for impingement to cause such a tear.

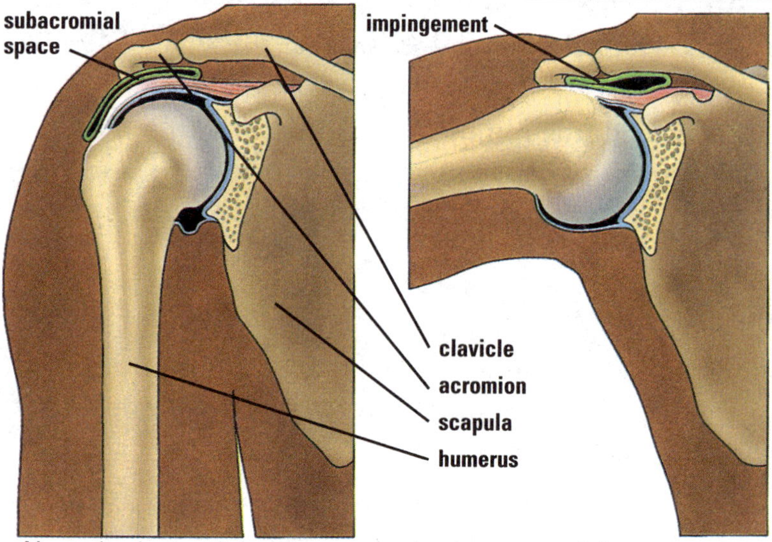

Normal subacromial space. Impingement of the rotator cuff.

The rubbing of the rotator cuff against the acromion can cause irritation to the tendons and **bursa**. The bursa is a thin sac of lubricating fluid that protects the rotator cuff and allows it to pass smoothly beneath the acromion. Inflammation of the bursa (**bursitis**) and of the tendons (**tendonitis**) may develop.

The tendonitis may come and go over several years. Calcium deposits may form. As a result, the rotator cuff may weaken and tear. Irregular bone growths, **bone spurs**, may also develop over time. They contribute to fraying and tearing of tendons that "catch" on them during arm movement.

Tears

As the rotator cuff becomes weakened by age, injury, postural strain, or repetitive motions, it can tear. Tears can spread both across and through the rotator cuff.

If the rotator cuff tear goes partially through the tendon, it is called a **partial-thickness tear**. Most often the rotator cuff tears away close to where it attaches to the humerus.

If the rotator cuff tear goes all the way through a tendon, it is called a **full-thickness** tear.

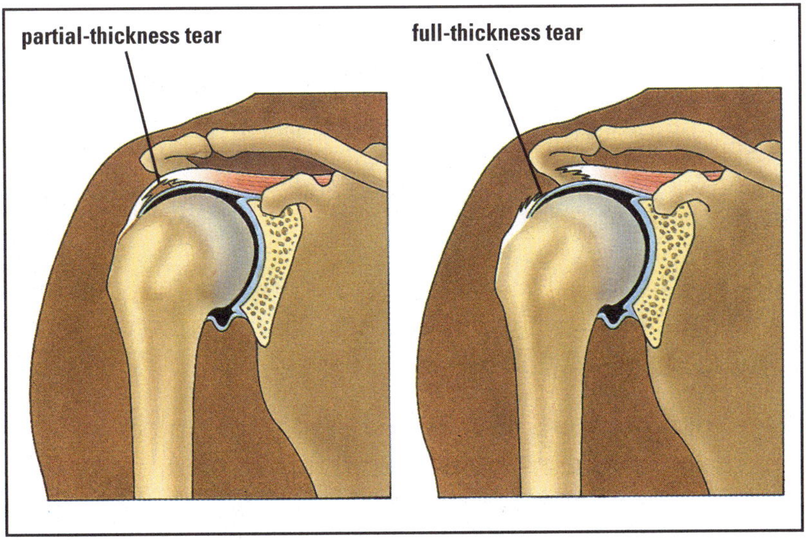

Indications of a Rotator Cuff Problem

Impingement and tears may feel the same and cause problems with the shoulder's function in a similar manner. Pain is usually felt in the front of the shoulder or on the outside part of the upper arm. Pain at night is common.

You may have trouble reaching for things, or using the arm overhead. The shoulder may make popping sounds, may feel as if it "catches," and may be weak.

EVALUATION FOR ROTATOR CUFF REPAIR

Up to 40 percent of people over 65 may have full-thickness rotator cuff tears without knowing it. Even a full-thickness rotator cuff tear may exist without symptoms of pain, weakness, or dysfunction.

Your physician may need to perform tests to tell whether there is impingement or a tear. Specific shoulder tests may include one or more of the following:

Impingement Test

An anesthetic is injected into the shoulder. If pain is no longer present during specific arm movements, then impingement may be present.

Steroids (cortisone) may be included in the injection to control any local inflammation which is causing pain.

X-rays

Shoulder x-rays may show whether the space between the acromion and head of the humerus (upper arm bone) is narrowed due to the shape of the acromion or bone spurs. X-rays can also detect bone fractures, joint dislocations, and arthritis.

Arthrogram

X-rays are taken after a small amount of dye is injected through a needle into the shoulder joint. The dye can be seen on x-ray and may help to show if a tear is present.

Ultrasound

Sound waves may sometimes be used to check for possible damage to the shoulder joint area.

MRI (Magnetic Resonance Imaging)

An MRI study uses a magnet and radio waves, along with a computer, to create many detailed images of the shoulder.

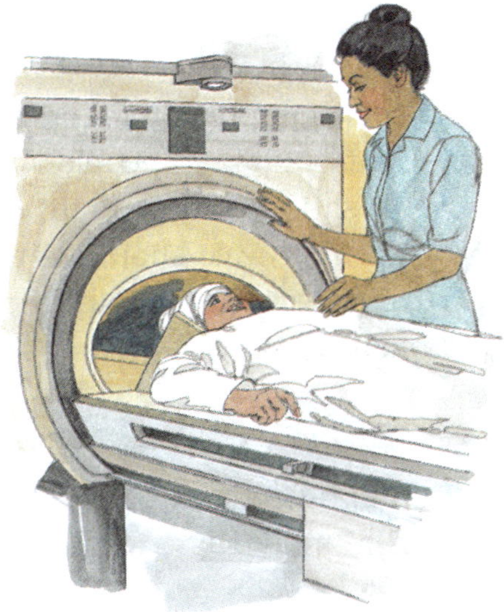

Tears and inflammation of rotator cuff tendons may show up on MRI.

Diagnostic Arthroscopy

A thin viewing tube is inserted into the joint through a small skin incision to check for rotator cuff tears directly. General or regional anesthesia is used.

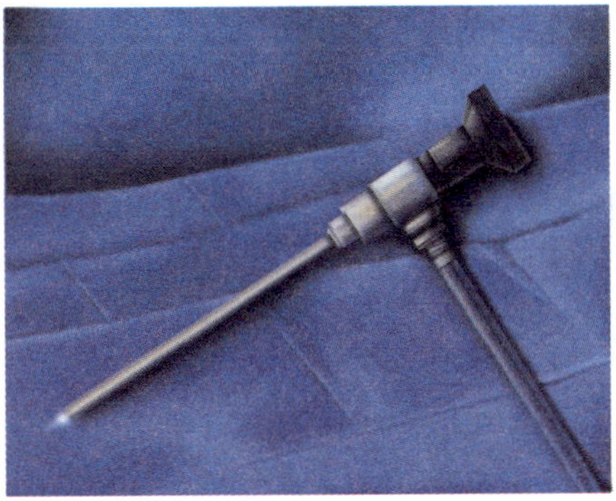

TREATMENT OPTIONS

Treatment options for impingement and rotator cuff injuries depend on the extent of the injury and how serious it is. The longer rotator cuff injuries go undiagnosed or untreated, the more difficult surgical treatment will be.

Most people with impingement can be treated without surgery. About half of the people with rotator cuff tears can recover a satisfactory amount of shoulder power, as well as a comfortable shoulder, without surgery. Non-surgical treatment includes therapeutic exercise, rest, and medications.

Pain from impingement or a rotator cuff tear may be controlled in many ways:

- Rest.
- Changing your activities.
- Anti-inflammatory medication.
- Ice packs or heat packs, or alternating both.
- Therapeutic exercises.
- Cortisone injections by your doctor.

For people over 65 who have had a tear for more than three months, non-surgical treatment may be advised.

WHEN IS SURGERY NEEDED?

If a program of conservative care cannot return the injured shoulder to less painful functioning, then rotator cuff repair or impingement relieving surgery is considered.

Rotator cuff repair is a surgical procedure to re-attach the torn tendon to the humerus. Proper healing requires that natural scar tissue form at the site of the repair to strengthen it.

Surgical repair may be considered for partial tears that extend more than halfway through a cuff tendon, and tears resulting from shoulder dislocation, fracture, or traumatic injury.

Rotator cuff repair may not be possible when the tear is too large, or when the tendon tissue is too weak.

If a favorable response to non-surgical treatment of impingement has not occurred within six months, surgery may be needed.

Rotator cuff repair is considered when:

- The tear results from injury, but the shoulder was normal before the injury.
- Pain remains unmanageable even with rest, therapeutic exercise, and medication.
- Weakness interferes with necessary tasks.

BEFORE SURGERY

Some standard tests are usually performed the week before surgery. These may include a chest x-ray, an **EKG (electrocardiogram)**, blood tests, and a urine test to make sure you are healthy enough for the surgery.

Going to the Hospital

People are usually admitted to the hospital on the day of the surgery. Occasionally, a person with diabetes, heart disease, or lung disease may be brought into the hospital the day before surgery.

Orthopedic surgeons work closely with nurses, physical therapists, and other health care professionals. All are part of a dedicated team to ensure the success of surgery.

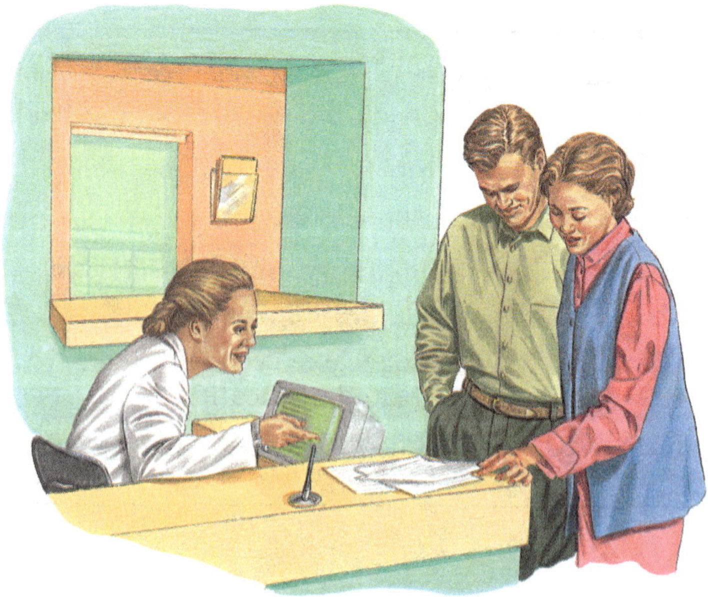

Inform your doctors about all the medications you are currently taking, including over-the-counter pain medications. Some medications may need to be stopped or adjusted the week or two before surgery. Also report any allergies you may have.

Anesthesia

Your surgeon or anesthesiologist will discuss with you the type of anesthesia to be used for your surgery.

Rotator cuff surgery is usually performed under **general anesthesia**, which will put you to sleep.

Some doctors and patients prefer **regional anesthesia**. With regional anesthesia, only the nerves that affect the arm and shoulder are numbed. Sedatives are also given for relaxation and comfort.

Do not eat or drink anything – not even a sip of water – during the eight hours before surgery. Anesthesia has fewer risks when the patient has an empty stomach. If you normally take medication during this time, consult your doctor about whether to take it on the day of surgery.

ROTATOR CUFF SURGERY

Impingement Surgery

When there is an ongoing problem with tendonitis and impingement of the cuff, a procedure called **subacromial decompression** may be recommended. This procedure creates more space for the rotator cuff.

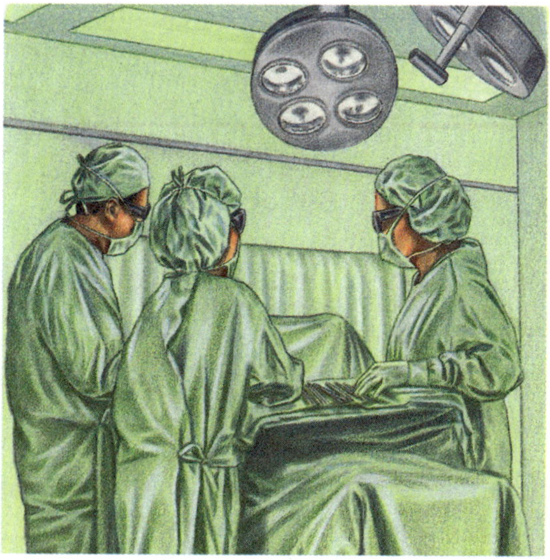

This surgery is done with the patient in a comfortable half-sitting position. An incision is made over the top of the shoulder. The deltoid muscle of the shoulder is opened. The underlying thickened bursa is removed. A tight ligament is often released from the acromion bone. The acromial bone spurs are removed and the shape of the normal bone is restored. The rotator cuff is then checked.

Rotator Cuff Repair

In addition to the steps taken for impingement-relieving surgery, the frayed edges of the torn rotator cuff are removed. Scar tissue is cut to restore tendon mobility.

The torn tendon is put back onto the humerus, if possible. Before the wound is closed, shoulder motion is checked to make sure that the repaired tendon will not pull away from the bone or rub against the acromion.

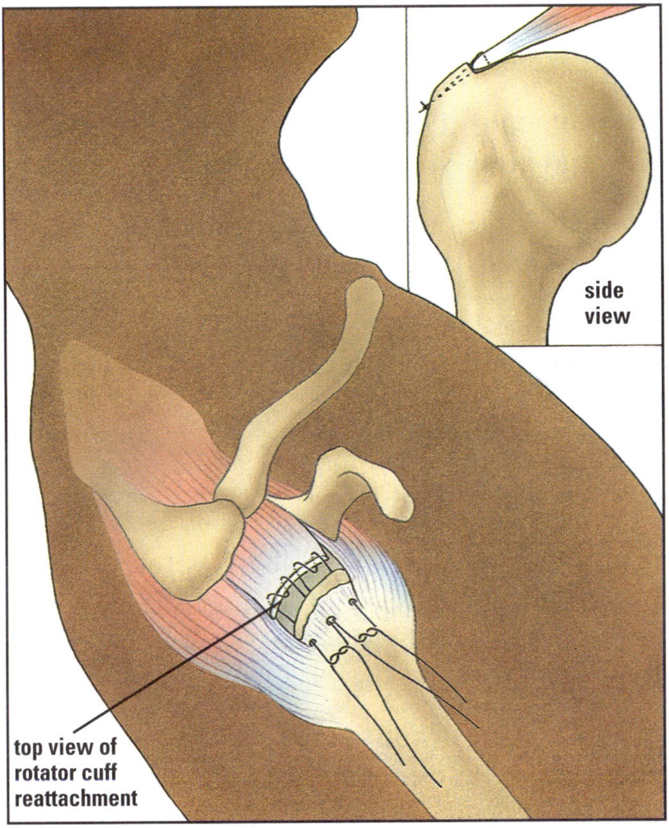

Side and top view of shoulder during rotator cuff repair.

Arthroscopy

A thin viewing tube (**arthroscope**) and other instruments can be inserted into the shoulder through very small skin incisions. Some surgeons prefer this technique for subacromial decompression and rotator cuff repair.

WHAT TO EXPECT AFTER SURGERY

After surgery, you will be taken to the recovery room with your arm in a sling, or perhaps, supported by a wedge-shaped pillow. You should be back in your room within two hours.

- An **intravenous (IV) line** in your arm or hand will deliver fluids and antibiotics directly into the bloodstream.
- You will be given a diet of clear liquids at first, followed later by solid food.

If you had general anesthesia, you will be given breathing exercises to counter its effects. Oxygen may be given if needed.

Managing Discomfort

The arm sling may be released to allow the elbow to straighten while lying down or sitting. The sling should not be removed. A cold pack or ice should be kept on the shoulder to reduce discomfort.

- For pain control, an injection at the base of the neck, called a **nerve block**, may be given to block the pain nerves to the shoulder and arm. You may have had a nerve block before surgery as well, to produce regional anesthesia.
- Pain medication may be given by mouth, injection in the muscle, or through the IV line.

Rehabilitation Therapy

While you are in the hospital, your therapist will visit you once or twice a day to help with exercises. You will be asked to exercise on your own as well.

The rehabilitation therapist acts as a coach and educator. Under your doctor's direction, the therapist will first teach you exercises to safely move your shoulder. Later, strengthening exercises will help return it to normal function.

Family members should meet the therapist while you are in the hospital to learn how they can help you once you are home.

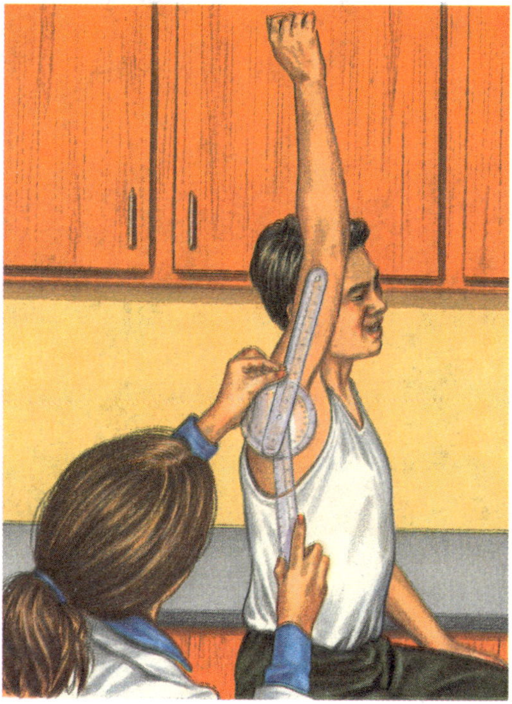

The rehabilitation therapist will work with you throughout your healing process to ensure that the best possible shoulder function is restored.

RECOVERY AT HOME

Most people return home the day after surgery. Some require an extra day in the hospital.

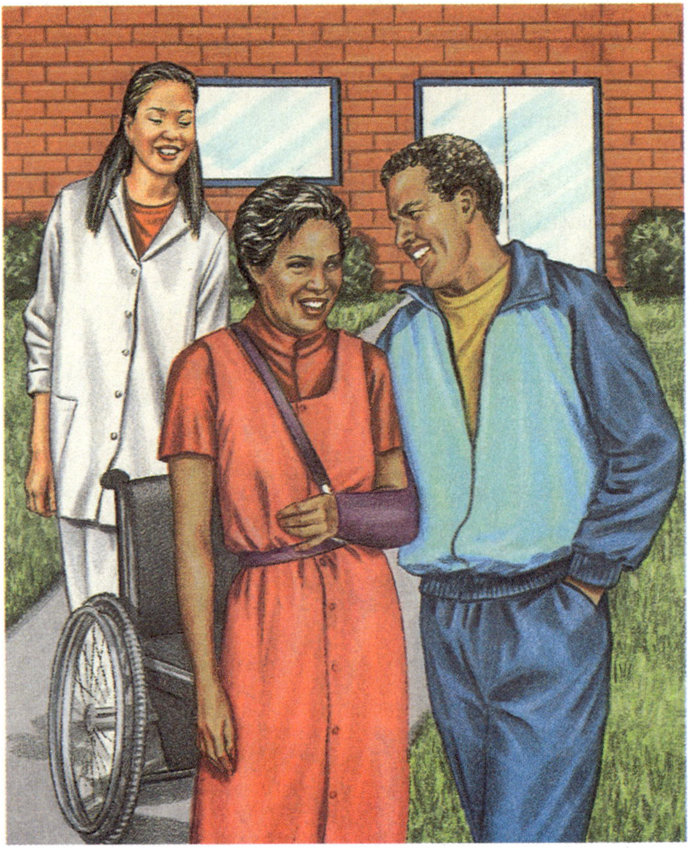

Caring For Your Shoulder

It is very important, except during therapeutic exercise, to strictly control the shoulder's activity for the first 12 weeks. Your sling is removed only for exercises and showering or bathing.

As much time as possible should be spent out of bed. You may shower when the intravenous line has been removed. Your bandage can be changed after the shower, if needed, or it may be discontinued.

Therapeutic exercises should be performed at home five times a day, or as recommended. After exercising, a cold pack or ice should be applied to the shoulder for comfort.

Bruising may appear in the skin surrounding the wound, or even in the arm below the wound. This is not cause for alarm. Also, the hand or forearm may swell. If this happens, elevate the arm and perform grip exercises until the swelling goes down. (See page 23.)

Call your doctor if the wound becomes red or warm, if fluid is draining from the wound, if you have a fever, or if you are bothered by pain.

INSTRUCTIONS FOR THE FIRST 12 WEEKS

Outside of the exercise sessions, you need to control the shoulder's activity strictly for the first 12 weeks.

Use the Sling

Wear the sling or brace at all times when walking. It may be released – but not removed – when sitting or lying awake in bed. It may be removed during exercise sessions. You may be advised to wear it while sleeping until near-normal arm control is regained.

Limit Use of the Arm

The arm and hand can be used for writing and eating, allowing for motion at the elbow and wrist only.

- **Do not push or pull.**
- **Do not use the arm for lifting.**
- **Do not reach forward or to the side.**

Showering

Once the wound is dry, you can shower without covering the wound, but arm support should be used, such as an old necktie looped around the neck and forearm.

Driving

Driving is not advised for the first 12 weeks. If a sudden stop or steering is required, you are likely to re-injure your shoulder.

The Follow-up Exam

A return visit with your surgeon will be made one to two weeks after surgery. The surgeon will check the wound and your shoulder's range of motion. Your doctor will answer any questions you have about exercises and activities.

Other visits will be scheduled as needed. Exercises will be added along the way, as your shoulder improves during the healing and rehabilitation period.

Rotator Cuff Exercises

Healing of the rotator cuff relies on scar tissue to bond the tendon attachment to bone. The healing process begins within six hours, but takes six to twelve months for complete healing. The shoulder needs to be protected during this time.

Therapy of the shoulder early on is important. It prevents scar tissue from forming in the wrong places.

- The goal is to safely regain maximum range of motion as soon as possible. This should take no more than one to three weeks.
- Exercise gently five times a day, or as instructed. Do 10 to 15 repetitions per exercise. Gradually increase the number of repetitions. Count to five while holding the position.

Do not perform exercises without consulting your surgeon or therapist.

BEGINNING EXERCISES

Gentle **range of motion** exercises are aimed at preventing stiffness from developing in the newly repaired shoulder.

Range of motion goals will be given with your exercise program. The following are some exercises for range of motion that may be recommended. Do these exercises gently, five times a day, or as recommended. Do each exercise 10 to 15 times.

Forward Elevation

Lie on your back. Keeping the elbow straight, raise the operated arm overhead with the aid of your uninjured arm (your "good" arm) or another person. Do not arch your back. **Do not rely on the muscles of the operated arm to do this exercise.**

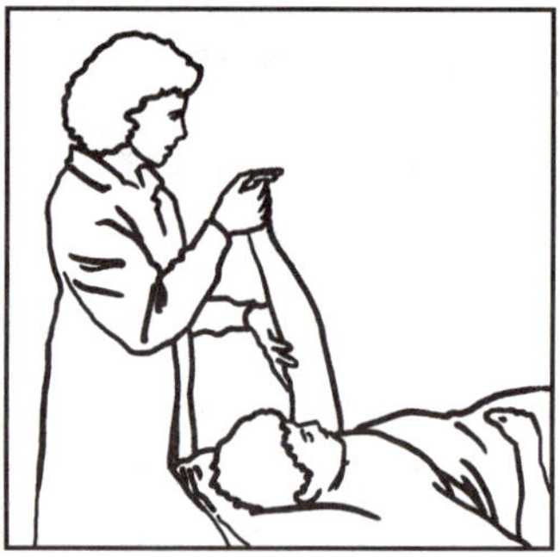

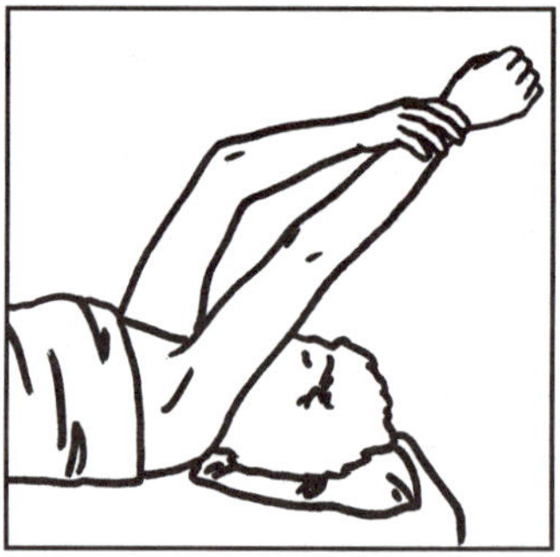

External Rotation

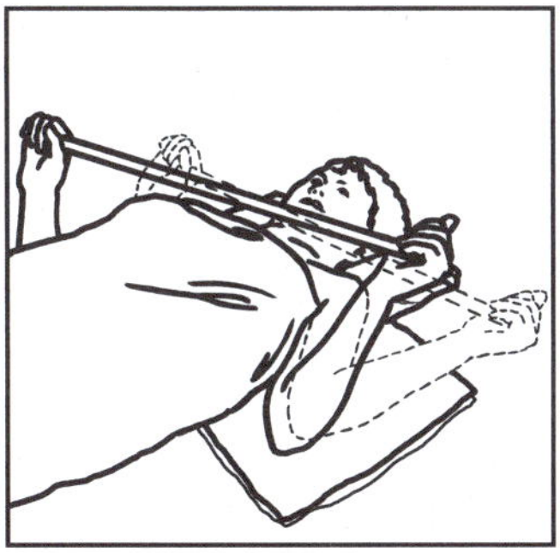

Lie on your back with a small pillow or folded towel beneath the elbow of the operated arm. Keep this elbow stable, close by your side at a 90 degree angle. Grasp a stick with both hands and use the "good" arm to push the operated arm out to the side until you feel a stretch.

Elbow Flexion and Extension

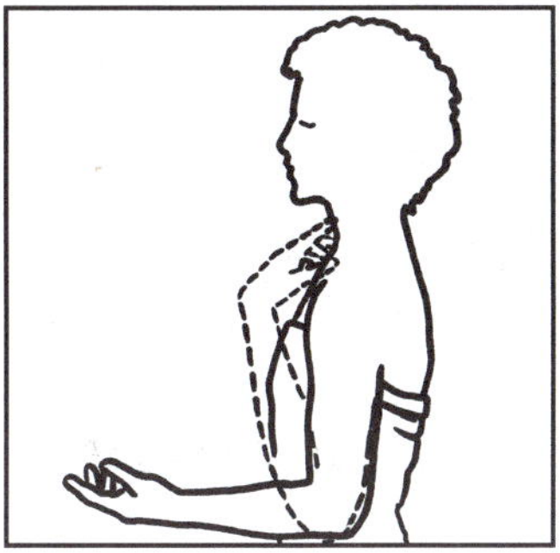

In a sitting position, bring your arm out of the sling. Flex and extend the elbow.

Grip Exercises

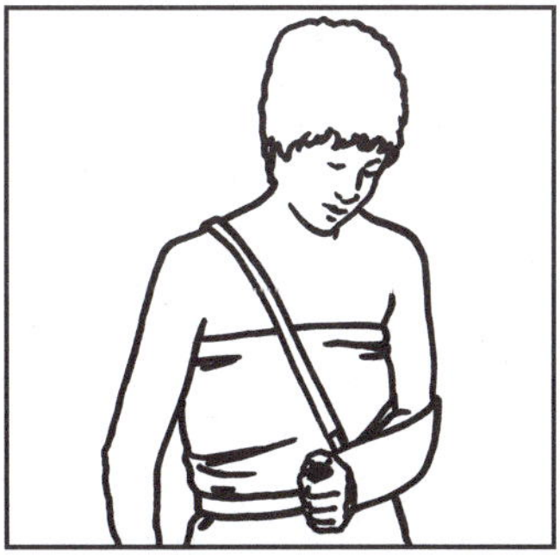

In a sitting position, practice squeezing a rubber ball. This helps maintain muscle power and reduce swelling.

No new exercises may be added for 8 to 12 weeks, depending on the size of the tear and the overall health of the rotator cuff.

LATER EXERCISES

Later exercises involve direct use of the shoulder muscles. These **active range of motion** exercises are begun about 12 weeks after surgery. Begin by doing the exercises gently, five times a day. Repeat each exercise 10 to 15 times to start. You will be given therapeutic exercise goals to work toward.

Stretching

Internal Rotation

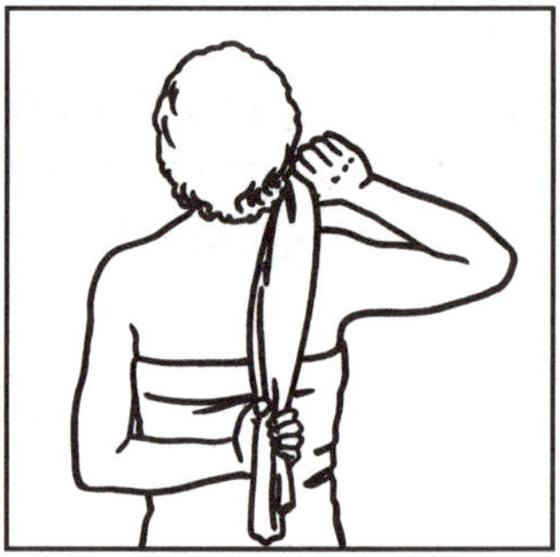

With your operated arm bent behind your back, move your thumb up and down along your backbone. You may use a towel to assist with this exercise, as shown.

Cross-Body Adduction

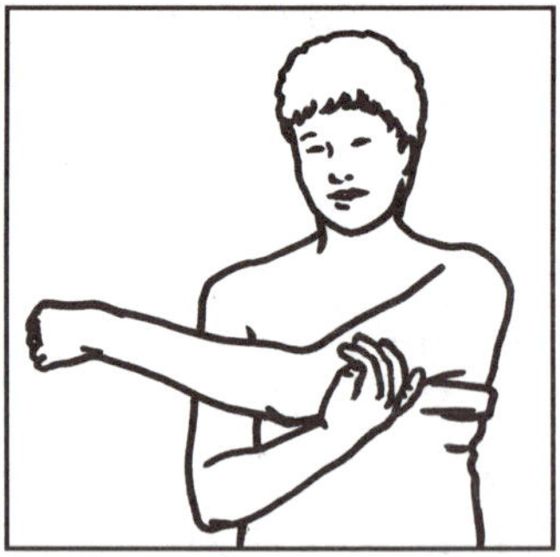

First hold your operated arm in front of you at shoulder level with the elbow relaxed. While in this position, bring your arm across the front of your body toward the uninjured shoulder. Use the good arm to assist.

Strengthening

External Rotation

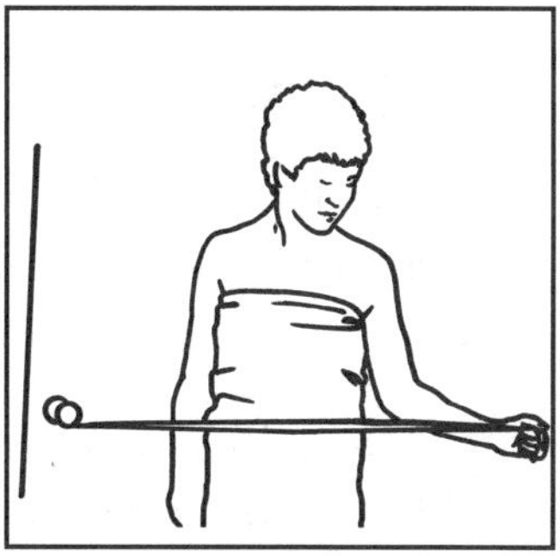

With the elbow of your operated arm close to your side and bent to a 90 degree angle, gently pull rubber exercise tubing, given to you by your physical therapist, in an outward direction.

Internal Rotation

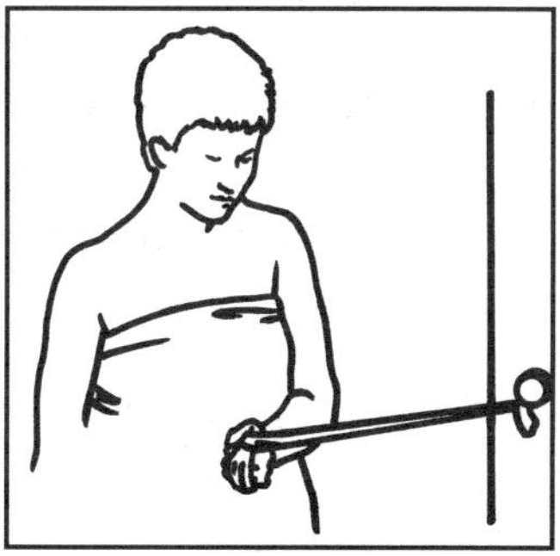

With your elbow close to your side and bent to a 90 degree angle, gently pull the rubber exercise tubing in an inward direction.

Pressing

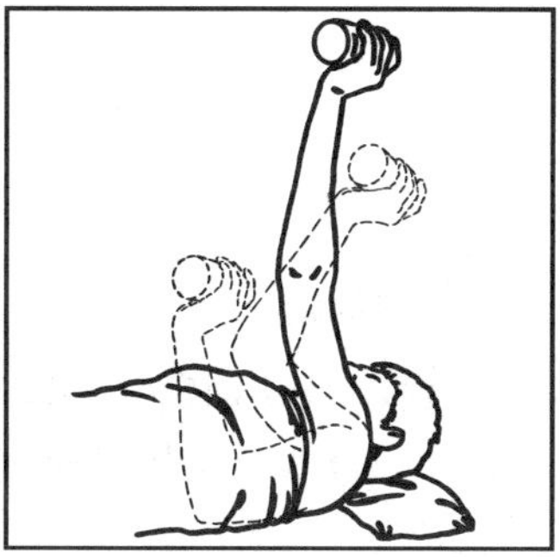

While lying on your back, push the hand of your operated arm straight up toward the ceiling while holding a light weight.

GETTING BACK TO NORMAL

Going Back to Work

When to go back to work depends on your occupation. You may be able to return to a sedentary or office job as early as one to two weeks after surgery.

Jobs involving heavy use of both arms will be difficult and can even endanger recovery. Manual tasks should be performed by the "good" arm only. Consult your doctor.

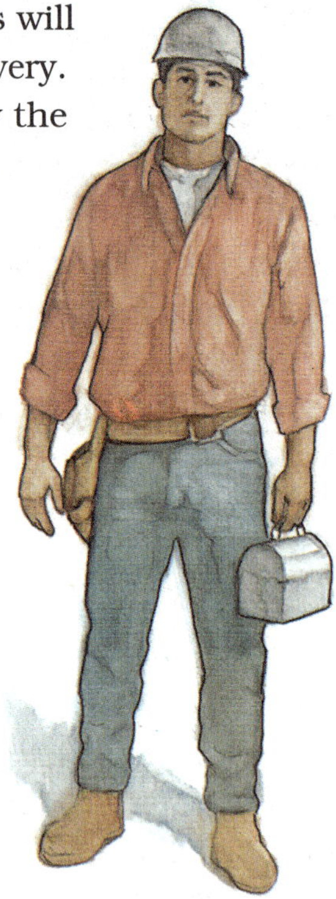

- If your job requires heavy use of both arms, you may have to wait up to six months before returning to work.
- Some types of work are not recommended following rotator cuff surgery. These include heavy manual labor involving lifting, climbing, or the use of heavy equipment.

Driving

You may usually start driving again three months after surgery.

Pain Relief

Within three to four weeks after surgery, the shoulder pain you originally had should be noticeably relieved. Early after the surgery, however, you will have pain from the surgery itself. This is normal and gradually disappears. There may be discomfort with exercise early on, especially during morning sessions.

It is important at this stage to manage the discomfort. Pain management includes over-the-counter medications to reduce inflammation and pain. Ice packs may also be useful.

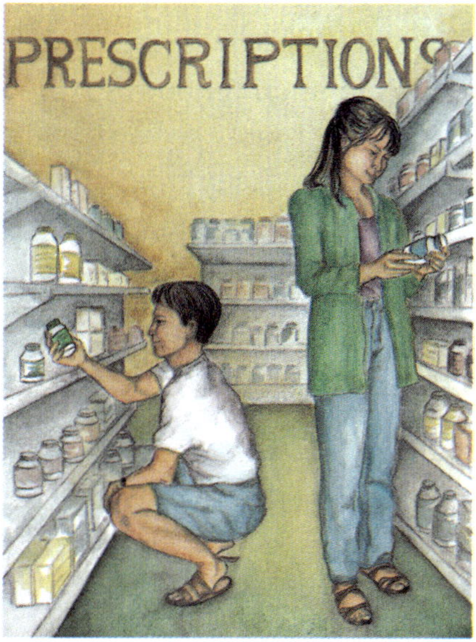

In combination with long-term exercises, pain management can help you recover flexibility and strength in your shoulder.

Staying with a Therapeutic Exercise Program

Therapeutic exercise is an important part of your recovery. A second surgery to repair a re-torn rotator cuff is much more difficult than the first repair. Additionally, 50 percent of re-torn rotator cuffs cannot be repaired.

Therefore, it is extremely important that your rehabilitation and exercise program is carefully followed.

When Is It Okay to Play Sports?

It is very important to avoid sports until the shoulder is properly healed. How soon you will be able to play sports depends on the size of the tear, how well your tendons are healing, and your progress in rehabilitation.

Walking is okay immediately after surgery, as long as a sling or brace is worn. Swimming is encouraged after three months, if your surgeon and therapist agree.

- Sports such as bowling or golf require at least four to six months of recovery. Golfers should move gradually back into the game. They should start with putting and chip shots, followed by gentle, short fairway shots and – much later – tee shots.
- Sports with sudden forceful movements, such as baseball, softball, tennis, or racquetball, require a minimum of six months recovery.
- Sports that may involve frequent falls (such as football and downhill skiing) should be avoided for at least one year.

Do not attempt any exercise or sports without consulting with your surgeon or rehabilitation therapist first.

Getting Back Into Sports After Surgery			
After 3 Months	**After 4 to 6 Months**	**After 6 Months**	**After 1 Year**
◆ Swimming ◆ Bicycling	◆ Racquetball ◆ Bowling ◆ Golf	◆ Baseball ◆ Tennis	◆ Football ◆ Downhill skiing ◆ Heavy weight lifting

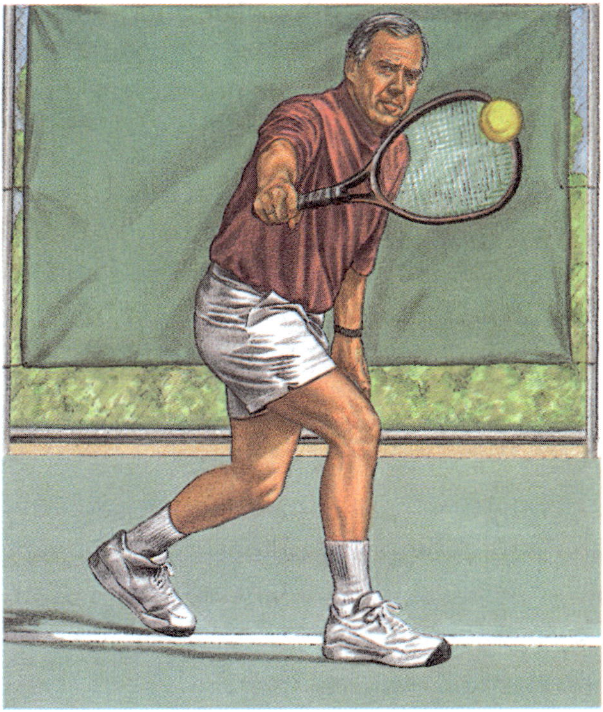

POSSIBLE COMPLICATIONS

Rotator cuff repair is a major surgical procedure. Most patients do very well and are pleased with the results. The potential for complications, however, should not be overlooked.

Stiffness

Stiffness can be a complication. The stiffness may have been present before surgery. More commonly, however, it develops when the shoulder is not exercised properly after surgery.

Stiffness that does not go away, even though you are following your therapeutic exercise program, may require more surgery. The surgeon may try to ease stiffness by moving the shoulder under anesthesia, or by removing scar tissue that may have formed.

Re-tear of the Rotator Cuff

Over-use of the arm or shoulder after surgery can re-tear the rotator cuff. A natural weakness in the tendon or bone may also cause the cuff to tear again.

Other Possible Complications

Some temporary numbness may occur at the incision site, but major nerve injury is unlikely. There is usually little bleeding with rotator cuff surgery.

SUMMARY

- The rotator cuff is a group of tendons that attach four short muscles of the shoulder blade to the upper arm bone. The rotator cuff helps stabilize and move the shoulder.
- The rotator cuff can weaken and tear as a result of injury, chronic strain, or age.
- In some cases of rotator cuff tear, comfort and function can be restored without surgery. Surgery may be necessary because of pain, loss of movement, or weakness.
- Full healing of the shoulder after surgery requires serious commitment to a therapeutic exercise program. This program emphasizes protection against re-injury. If the therapeutic exercise program is not followed, stiffness may develop or the cuff may tear again.
- Exercises to recover strength and flexibility are added gradually as the shoulder heals.
- Normal daily activities, work, and sports are also added by your surgeon or therapist at regular intervals from the time of surgery, depending on how well the shoulder is healing and whether there are any complications.
- Complications after surgery can include temporary numbness, stiffness, and re-tear of the rotator cuff.

GLOSSARY

Acromion
A specific part of the shoulder blade (scapula) that is located above the rotator cuff.

Arthroscopy
A surgical procedure in which a thin viewing tube and other instruments are inserted through small incisions. Arthroscopy can sometimes be used instead of open surgery for subacromial decompression, and to repair the rotator cuff.

Bone spurs
Irregular bone growths that may be removed during surgery.

Bursitis
Inflammation of the lubricating sac of fluid (bursa) in the shoulder joint.

Humerus
The upper arm bone.

Full-thickness tear
A rotator cuff tear that goes all the way through a tendon.

Impingement
A shoulder disorder that results from a narrowing of the space beneath the acromion that may lead to irritation, inflammation, weakness, and tearing of the rotator cuff.

Partial-thickness tear
A rotator cuff tear that goes partially through a tendon.

Rotator cuff
A group of four tendons that connect four muscles of the shoulder blade to the upper arm bone (humerus).

Subacromial decompression
Surgery to increase the space around the rotator cuff when impingement is a problem.

Tendons
Tough, stringy bands of tissue at the ends of muscles that connect the muscles to the bones.

Tendonitis
Inflammation of the tendons.